I0447098

The Secret Fountain of Youth

By Jon Michael Caravella

ISBN: 1475175736
ISBN-13: 978-1475175738

The Secret Fountain of Youth

Contents

Chapters

Introduction

The information in this book might be shocking to some readers. My intentions are not to tear down our medical society, it's to help people. This is not meant to be an attack against anyone or any organization. What I found might be the World's best kept secrets. It could just be the most forbidden secret of the medical world.

In my research, I read that fungus, and bacteria are the main causes of our bodies breaking down and getting sick. What if we could eliminate a lot of these things that are making us sick from our lives? What if we could stay well most of the time? Keep fungus and bacteria under control in our bodies, so we don't get sick as often? Life would be much more pleasant, don't you think?

All of the information in this book is scattered throughout the World Wide Web. I did not make it up; I just kept asking my computer research questions and there it was, a man-made chemical that is making us and the whole world very sick—and you won't believe what it is. It just took someone like me to put all the pieces together in one place and look at the whole picture.

Then I found the one natural thing that can make us better. It's what some people call the Fountain of Youth. I have it right here nestled in Florida, and I call it The Secret Fountain of Youth. It's been right in front of us for years and years; some people know of it already and use it all the time. No one was hiding it from us. It has always been right there in front of our eyes, at arm's reach, and lots of people have written about it. But no one had all the pieces in order to paint the picture I have painted.

You see, I have psoriasis and psoriatic arthritis, and I had been searching the World Wide Web for years, hoping to find out what psoriasis really is, what causes it, and how I could clear it up.

I asked my doctor a few questions and she gave me her best answers. One of my questions was whether chlorine, the chemical acid, could be causing my psoriasis? She smiled and said, "Maybe, and you could also be having an allergic reaction to stainless steel. Try taking an allergy pill and keep searching," with a smile on her face. I knew then I was close to finding the secret—it was just a matter of time.

I now knew that psoriasis is an allergic reaction to something, but what? Then I thought about what many other doctors have told me over the years. Psoriasis is a hereditary disease. I found out they were not kidding about that part—it's true. I inherited an overactive immune system from my dad.

That is the system that does not like whatever it is that's contacting or going into my body. This came from my dad because he also had psoriasis.

Then I read that psoriasis was just a plutonic name for a skin conditions like eczema and dermatitis; in fact, the word psoriasis is Greek for "*itchy*." They're right: it gets very itchy and painful, and it bleeds when you scratch it.

I had been searching for years for a cure, and one day I put it all my research together and found the missing link. Not only did I find the cause of psoriasis, but I found the source that was making us sick. Yes sick—like colds, flu, arthritis, gout, kidney stones, to name a few. It has been confirmed by several doctors that psoriasis is caused by exposure to the environment.

I started breaking out with psoriasis for the first time in Southern California, when they first introduced chloramine in to the reservoirs, and it killed all the fish in the reservoirs. The day after they put chloramine in the reservoirs, I broke out with little bumps on my scalp. Then little by little, patches developed on my body. Chloramine causes an allergic reaction when it gets on my skin. *I found the cause to my psoriasis!* I thought.

Then I searched the chemical properties that make up chloramine, and you won't believe what I found: the true answer to one of the things I am allergic to. It's not just the possible cause of my psoriasis, but the hidden secret to sickness in our bodies and what's making our planet sick.

It's what I believe killed the blackbirds and is confusing the mammals in the oceans. It's making acid rain and is killing our ozone layer. It's possibly making our children sick.

Now I am not a doctor or a scientist and I know this is a very strong claim, but I can back it all up with where and how I came up with my conclusion.

All the information in this book was found on the World Wide Web. I have provided links in this book to

where I found a lot of the information. Lots of people have done wonderful research that helped me put the puzzle together. I thank them for their great research work.

I have made up nothing; it all came off the World Wide Web, and I connected the pieces and put the puzzle together to see the big picture. You will understand more of my claim as you read on.

I will take you piece by piece to show you the picture that I have found; then you can decide for yourself.

Check out more info on Psoriasis at:

http://psoriasis.about.com/lw/Health-Medicine/Alternative-treatments/Psoriasis-and-Itching.h

Chapter One

What is Gout and Arthritis?

Gout occurs when the body is producing too much uric acid or the kidneys are not able to properly eliminate all the uric acid from the urine. Uric acid is a byproduct of cells breakdown, and because the body is continually breaking down and forming new cells, uric acid is commonly present in small amounts in the bloodstream. The body also breaks down a substance in foods known as purine into uric acid. When you have too much uric acid in your body, it turns into uric acid crystals and stored in your joints and tissue.

This can cause intense and sudden inflammation, pain, redness, stiffness, and burning in and around joints where it's stored. Gout can persist for several weeks or even months. Gout often starts in one of the big toes, but it can also affect the fingers, wrists, elbows, knees, ankles, heels, and other joint areas.

This will also shock you: some doctors are now calling some forms of arthritis "gouty arthritis," but I call it uric acid poisoning. Gout is most commonly seen in men forty and up, but it can strike anyone at any age, especially postmenopausal women, it can even strike children.

Serious complications of gout are kidney stones and/or gallstones. Whether it's rheumatoid arthritis, psoriatic arthritis, or just gouty arthritis, they all do the same thing: damage our joints and cause pain. Some arthritis is caused by too much uric acid in our bodies. Some of the pain is from the bones that have thinned over time from low potassium levels and loss of cartilage in the joints. Some arthritis is from dehydration caused by medicine given to us for water buildup. Other conditions, or just lack of nutrition, either way, it's painful.

More on this at:

http://en.wikipedia.org/wiki/Gout

http://arthritis.emedtv.com/gout/gouty-arthritis.html

Causes of Gout and Arthritis

Normally uric acid is broken down in the blood and eliminated in your urine. When the body increases its production of uric acid and the kidneys cannot eliminate enough uric acid from the body, the blood reaches a saturation point.

At that point the body is unable to eliminate enough uric acid, so it deposits a hardened crystallized form of uric acid, usually in the joint fluid and the joint lining.

Although in extreme cases, uric acid crystals can affect many of the body's joints and damage the kidneys. Purines waste and uric acid is usually cleared from the system through the kidneys by way of the urine. In extreme cases arthritis can affect many of the body's joints and damage the kidneys.

However sometimes your body can produce too much uric acid, or there might be a problem with the kidneys clearing out all of the uric acid in our body's. That's when you get uric acid crystals forming and building up in your body's.

Read more at:

http://wiki.answers.com/Q/Why_does_uric_acid_accumulate_in_joints

http://www.gout.com/causes-triggershttp://www.whathealth.com/gout/causes.html

Chapter Two

Gout and Arthritis Symptoms

Gout is a form of arthritis; it causes inflammation and swelling of the joints and is caused by the buildup of uric acid in the body. Certain foods cause gout, so diet plays a big role. The most common gout symptom is a sudden attack of pain, tenderness, redness, warmth, and swelling in some joints. It usually affects one joint at a time, especially the joint of the big toe, but it can also affect the knee, ankle, foot, hand, wrist and elbows.

We need a certain amount of ammonia that comes from our food, just cut back on the amount of man-made ammonia; this will be a good starting point.

I know it will take time for the uric acid crystals to dissolve—that does not happen overnight. Also I am not sure if the damage that has already been done in your bodies is reversible. But I do know our bodies were made to heal themselves when our pH is balanced.

Treatment of gout can be achieved through proper diet. Eliminate as much, man-made acid as possible from getting in or onto our body's each day. Read labels on boxes, look for ammonia in them, and cut back from using it so much. I am not telling you to stop using ammonia product completely; that would be totally impossible— ammonia is everywhere just cut back.

Foods that Cause Gout

You will benefit from a reduction of purine-rich foods. These include beer and other alcoholic beverages, anchovies, sardines (in oil), fish roe, herring, yeast, organ meats, liver, kidneys, legumes (dried beans, peas, and soybeans), meat extracts, consommé, gravies, mushrooms, spinach, asparagus, cauliflower, poultry, and some juices.

Weight loss can also help reduce uric acid levels in the body of people that are overweight. If you go on an alkaline diet, you will start losing weight naturally once your pH level gets normal. Take a look at the chart below to find the level of acidity in your favorite foods and drinks:

Foods with very high purine levels (up to 1,000 mg per 3.5 ounce serving): anchovies, brains, gravies, gravies, kidneys, sardines, sweetbreads.

Food with moderately low to high and purine levels (5-100 mg per 3.5 ounce serving). Asparagus, bacon, beef, bluefish, bouillon, calf tongue, chicken, chicken soup, codfish, duck, goose, halibut, ham, kidney beans, lamb, lentils, lima beans, lobster, mushrooms, mutton, navy beans, oatmeal, oysters, peas, perch, pork, rabbit, salmon, shellfish, snapper, spinach, tripe, trout, tuna, turkey, veal, and venison.

This link is to a download from the FDA on the approximate pH levels of foods and food products. This will help you a lot with knowing what is too acidic and what is not.

Read more at:

http://www.pronamel.us/pdfs/FDA%20pH%20of%20Foods%20April%202007-optimized.pdf

I have a question for you, If you had cancer and your doctor gave you six months to live, and you found out if you adjust your pH to a 7.0–7.2 balance by taking ACV, that it could possibly clear up your cancer, would you not do everything in your power to get some and try it?

Then

------------ **WHY WAIT?** -----------

Preventive medicine is a better way to stay healthy and keep from getting sick.

I'm not a doctor so I cannot tell you if this will work for you. But I read on the World Wide Web that for thousands of years, many people and many societies have claimed it has worked for them. If I had cancer or any other sickness, or disease and a doctor told me there was no known cure for it, I would definitely give everything including apple cider vinegar a try. I would not go out without a fight.

Our bodies are being bombarded by too much *MAN-MADE AMMONIA*. It's causing a high buildup of uric acid in our bodies. Man-made ammonia in high quantities is also making the earth and everything on it very sick. Something needs to be done now, or the future will be grim for us and Mother Earth.

Here are some other links that I found interesting:

http://www.eatingbirdfood.com/2012/02/health-benefits-of-apple-cider-vinegar-acv/

http://www.pronamel.us/what_is_acid_erosion/food_acidity_finder.aspx?bing=b_&rotation=3672&banner=24911&kw=306450-

Uric Acid Crystals

Definition: Uric acid: is the final product of purine metabolism in human beings.

Deposits of uric acid can appear as lumps under the skin around the joints and at the rim of the ear. In addition, uric acid crystals can also collect in the kidneys and cause kidney stones. That's the worst pain a guy can go through—it's like having a baby, and you feel like you had one once you passed that stone. Once you do pass one, you never ever want to go through that pain again.

Uric acid crystals also build up in your gallbladder and make help make gallstones, which usually require an operation. I read if you start using apple cider vinegar with mother it will dissolve the crystals. I think if I had an attack of gallstones, I would try apple cider vinegar first before having an operation.

I was watching the news the other day; and a story about some teenage girls that go to the same school, are coming down with a Tourette like syndrome. I could not help think how much that problem sounds like what I am talking about in this book. I think if I were their dad or mom, I would check to see what they are using for hygiene products, and if they contain ammonia. I would also check what they are eating, and also what the school is using for cleaning products. I believe there may be a possible link to what I am sharing with you in this book.

Uric acid concentrations, both above and below normal levels, have been linked to a number of diseases. I also found on the web, that an abnormally high uric acid level has been linked with, hypertension, cardiovascular disease, and renal disease.

This has also been documented: An abnormally high concentration level of uric acid, have been linked to multiple sclerosis, Parkinson's disease, Alzheimer's disease, and optic neuritis disease. Historically, uric acid has been considered a marker of these disease states.

Recent studies have provided evidence that uric acid levels may actually play a role in the development and or progression of such diseases. As a result, uric acid concentrations are now either included in, or being investigated for, the treatment of a variety of disease states.

More on this at:

http://jpet.aspetjournals.org/content/324/1/1.long

The Secret Fountain of Youth

Chapter Three
What is Acidosis or an Acidic Body?

Acidosis or an acidic body is when your body is out of balance and the pH level is low due to an accumulation of waste matter in the system (uric acid). Usually an acidic body tries to excrete toxins through *bowel movements*, *skin eruptions*, and *urination.*

On occasions, due to poor elimination of toxins, uric acid crystals accumulate in our bodies over time. The average diet consists mainly of acid-forming foods, the causes of excess uric acid in our bodies. The excess get stored in the form of uric acid crystals.

Some others ways we take in ammonia are through grooming products and cleaning products along with our meats and chicken packing-houses. They are adding a lot of ammonia to our daily intake, causing high levels of uric acid in our bodies. Eating these acid-forming foods will cause uric acid in your system to build up, resulting in a low acidy pH level and long-term health concerns.

Among the male population in the United States, approximately five million men suffer from gout. Others suffer from kidney stones and other diseases, but most will suffer from arthritis as they age. That's because uric acid levels and uric acid crystals build up over time in different parts of our bodies.

This will lead to arthritis and gout somewhere in our bodies; everyone is different. Other causes of an over-acidic body may include commercial fertilizers, shampoos, skin, body, and hair care products, household detergents, lawn pesticides, drinking water, Freon, acid rain, chlorides, and chloramine, to name a few.

(Did you know that none other than Benjamin Franklin had terribly painful gouty arthritis?)

Gout is nine times more common in men than in women. It predominantly attacks males after puberty, with a peak age of seventy-five. In women, gout attacks usually occur after menopause. An elevated blood level of uric acid may indicate an increased risk of gout. There are some people with repeated gout attacks that have normal uric-acid blood levels when checked.

Read more on this at:

http://en.wikipedia.org/wiki/Anhydrous_ammonia

What are Purines?

Purines are natural substances found in all of the body's cells and in virtually all foods. The reason for their widespread occurrence is simple. Purines provide a part of the chemical structure of our genes and the genes of plants and animals. A relatively small number of foods contain concentrated amounts of purines. For the most part these high-purine foods are also high-protein foods. They include organ meats like kidney, fish like mackerel, herring, sardines and mussels, and also yeast. Uric acid is the chemical formed when purines have been broken down completely.

It's normal and healthy for uric acid to be formed in the body from the breakdown of purines. In our blood, for example, uric acid serves as an antioxidant it helps prevent damage to our blood-vessel linings. A continual supply of uric acid is important for protecting our blood vessels.

However to high Uric acid levels in the blood and other parts of the body can become overwhelming to our kidneys, under a variety of circumstances. Since our kidneys are responsible for helping keep blood levels of uric acid balanced, kidney problems can lead to excessive accumulation of uric acid in various parts of the body.

Excessive breakdown of cells can also cause uric acid build up. When uric acid accumulates, uric acid crystals can become deposited in our tendons, joints, kidneys, and other organs. This accumulation of uric acid crystals is called gouty arthritis, or simply "gout."

Read more on purines at:

http://www.livestrong.com/article/32170-purines/

There are places in this book where I repeat myself, I did this so you can get a good understanding of what I am trying to show you.

Also check out the world's healthiest foods at:

http://www.whfoods.com/genpage.php?tname=george&dbid=51

What is Hyperuricemia?

Definition: hy·per·u·ri·ce·mi·a An unusually high concentration of uric acid in the blood.

Hyperuricemia: is the present state of excess uric acid in the body's blood products

Hyperuricemia is not a disease but it is dangerous to our bodies. Several illnesses, such as hyperthyroidism or an excessive level of thyroid hormones in the body, can cause hyperuricemia.

It may also be caused by inflammation of the kidneys, called nephritis. Those with multiple sclerosis may be prone to hyperuricemia, and as well, people with bone marrow cancer may be at risk also.

People who are fed intravenously may also be at risk for high uric acid content. Certain medications like allopurinol, which is used to treat gout, as well as excessive consumption of alcohol or alcoholism, may also cause hyperuricemia. High levels of fructose, the sugars from fruit and fruit juices, can also result in the condition.

Hyperuricemia can be the causal factor for several conditions. High concentrates of uric acid can lead to kidney or bladder stones, which then either must be painfully passed or surgically removed.

The kidneys turn uric acid into urate in a healthy, normal body with no underlying problems. Approximately 70 to 75 percent of the urate produced daily is excreted by the kidneys, while the rest is eliminated by the intestines. This is the Statistics of a healthy normal body with no underlying problems.

Read more on this at:

http://www.arthritis.about.com/od/gout/g/hyperuricemia.htm

http://www.wisegeek.com/what-is-hyperuricemia.htm

I recommend getting

some pH test paper from your health food store,

or you can order them online;

just do a search.

Test yourself and your loved ones

twice a day, morning and night,

and keep a log.

Once you know your body's pH level is OK,

then test it weekly to keep it in range.

If you start feeling sick check,

your pH and keep track of your numbers

Chapter Four

The Arthritis Foundation Claims

The Arthritis Foundation claims that uric acid levels are not the only causes of gout attacks: They claim a gout attack can also be triggered by the following:

1. Joint injury, surgery, or sudden illness:

This is because blood circulation is what moves the uric acid to the kidneys and then flushes it out of our bodies. Joint injury can cause slow blood circulation due to swelling. Surgery and/or sudden illness can cause dehydration in your body, which cases uric acid buildup also.

2. Taking certain medications for high blood pressure, leg swelling, or heart failure:

This is because certain medications like water pills for high blood pressure and incontinence pills can and do cause dehydration in your body and a buildup of uric acid. Also, some medicines have ammonia or alcohol in them and ammonia and alcohol turns to uric acid in our bodies.

3. Crash diets and fasting:

This is because diets high in protein make too much acid in our bodies, causing high levels of uric acid. Lack of water in our bodies from not eating right from crash diets and dehydration keeps your kidneys from flushing out uric acid properly.

4. Dehydration from meds and diarrhea:

This is because we need at least eight glasses of

water a day to flush out uric acid from your kidneys; less can cause a

buildup of uric acid in our bodies.

5. Drinking too much alcohol:

This is because alcohol also causes dehydration; this causes uric acid to build up in our bodies

6. Drinking sweet sodas:

This is because there is phosphoric acid in soda and soda does not replace water loss in our bodies. This causes dehydration and uric acid build up in our bodies.

7. Eating foods high in purines:

This is because purines are natural substances found in all of the body's cells and virtually in all our foods. Purines are metabolized into uric acid. Too much man-made ammonia turns to uric acid causes uric acid crystals in our bodies.

All of these ailments listed above can cause dehydration and/or diarrhea and can cause gout and arthritis. This is because your body must stay within a pH range of 7.0 to 7.5.

The term **"arthritis"** encompasses more than a hundred diseases and conditions that affect the joints in our bodies. The word "arthritis" is just a generic term. Approximately forty-six million Americans have some type of arthritis or related condition.

Read more on this at

http://www.arthritis.org/women.php

Chapter Five

What is Ammonia?

Ammonia is a colorless gas with a very sharp odor, made both by man and by nature. The amount of man-made ammonia produced every year is equal to that produced by nature every year. Ammonia is produced naturally in soil by bacteria, by decaying plants and animals, and by animal wastes. It's also man-made in some factories around the world.

Ammonia can be irritating; if you are exposed to high concentrations in the air, it can severely burn your skin, eyes, throat, and lungs.

Pure ammonia is sometimes referred to as anhydrous ammonia to distinguish it from aqueous solutions of ammonia. For example, household ammonia is actually a solution of at least 90 percent water and less than 10 percent ammonia (NH_3). Ammonia has many applications and is one of the most commonly manufactured inorganic chemicals. Anhydrous ammonia is prepared commercially from natural gas, air, and steam.

Check out this website for the Department of Health and Senior Services:

http://web.doh.state.nj.us/rtkhsfs/factsheets.aspx?lan=english&alph=A&carcinogen=False&new=False

Where is Ammonia in the World?

Liquid ammonia is found in many household cleaners. Also, eggs are dunked in to ammonia to kill bacteria that may be on them. Our meats are also getting a bath with ammonia; Meat packing houses use it to collect the slime and put it back into the meat so they get less waste—and the FDA told them it's OK to do that.

An estimated ten trillion gallons a year of untreated storm water runs off roofs, roads, parking lots, and other paved surfaces. It travels through the sewage systems, into our rivers, waterways and reservoirs that serve as our drinking water supplies. It also drains in to out rivers and streams and in to the ocean. Increasing health risks and degrading ecosystems, as direct result.

Animal, birds, and fishes also deposit uric acid in to our world as they relieve themselves. Oh, and let's not forget acid rain. Animal waste from large factories and farms is threatening our health, and even the water we drink and swim in. As you can see, ammonia is all around us and man-made ammonia is threatening the future of our nation's rivers, lakes, and streams.

Ammonia is essential for many biological processes. Most of the ammonia produced in chemical factories is used to make fertilizers. The remaining ammonia is used in textiles, plastics, explosives, pulp and paper production, food and beverages, household cleaning products, refrigerants, cosmetics, and other products. It is also used in smelling salts. Check everything you use and eat in your homes, see if it contains ammonia.

To read more check out:

http://www.encyclopedia.com/topic/water_pollution.aspx

Names they use for Ammonia are

anhydrous ammonia, ammonium hydroxide, ammonium sulfate, ammonium chloride, Sal ammoniac, NH_4Cl, crystalline salt, hydrochloric acid, anionic surfactant, alkyl sulfate, lauryl sulfates, potassium lauryl sulfate, sodium laureth sulfate, sodium lauryl sulfate, sodium nitrate, 2NH3, 4NH3, NH3, ammonium hydroxide, and ammonia.

Read more on this at:

http://www.nrdc.org/water/pollution/cesspools/execsum.

Ammonia Allergies and Reactions

Have you ever had strange allergic reactions or symptoms like these after visiting your hairdresser? Eczema of the scalp, itchy, watery eyes, coughing, sneezing or scalp burns?

You may have had an allergic reaction to ammonia or alcohol. That's because most hair-coloring products contain one or the other. You can use Organic Color Systems to solve the problem, ask your hairstylist about them.

Check out the link below.

http://www.puresouthport.com/page1.php

Skin reactions to ammonia and/or alcohol include dry skin, eczema, redness, hives, itching, swelling, and blisters. Ammonia causes symptoms associated with allergic rhinitis, conjunctivitis, and asthma such as runny nose, itchy and watery eyes, sneezing, wheezing, shortness of breath, and coughing. In extreme cases, blindness, lung damage, or death can occur from concentrated dosages of ammonia or alcohol.

Breathing lower concentrations dosages of either ammonia or alcohol can cause itchy, watery eyes, wheezing, sneezing, shortness of breath and coughing. Ammonia dissolves easily in water and evaporates quickly. Some of the rockets we shoot in to space use ammonia chloride (ammonium chloride is a rocket fuel).

Our fertilizer is also ammonium chloride, and plants breaking down and decomposing makes ammonia.

Read more on ammonia allergies at
http://www.ehow.com/facts_6319581_ammonia-allergies.html

What is Pink Slime?

Back in 1990 the FDA approved the use of ammonia in our meat packing houses. Some large packing houses use ammonia to clean the slug off the tables, and for cleaning the scrap of meat and fat they pick up off the floor and then use the slug as fillers in our hamburger, pork and chicken meat.

They also use ammonia to disinfect the meat. That's why meat does not have flavor like it did a long time ago. The meat today has very little flavor and has a faint smell of ammonia. They are also taking paces of meat they would normally toss out and soak it in ammonia; as a result, it's as tender as sirloin but it not good for us to eat.

Once only used in dog food and cooking oil, the beef trimmings are now sprayed with ammonia so they are safe to eat and added to most ground beef as cheaper filler.

Seventy percent of the ground beef we buy at the supermarket contains something they call "pink slime" (*AMMMONIA*).

Read more on this at

http://www.reuters.com/article/2012/04/04/us-food-ammonia-idUSBRE8331B420120404

http://lisamurphy.weebly.com/final-collaborative-research-project.html

(Are you seeing the Picture Yet?)

You know, I would not be a bit surprised if they are doing the same to our veggies. How about our milk—have you noticed that if you leave your milk in the refrigerator past the expiration date and smell it a month later, it still smells and it tastes like you just opened it up fresh? I wonder if they are doing something with that also.

Some more good reading at:

http://www.notmilk.com/

http://www.sumobrain.com/patents/wipo/Process-preparation-deacidified-coffee/WO1996028038.htm

Cigarettes and Ammonia

During the 1960s, tobacco companies such as Brown & Williamson and Philip Morris began using *ammonia* in cigarettes. They found that ammonia reinforces the **_addictive ability_** and flavor of nicotine.

Read more on this at:

http://tobaccodocuments.org/landman/00044858-4879.html

Cigarettes Contain Polonium-210

Tobacco companies knew that cigarettes contained a radioactive substance called Polonium-210, but hid that knowledge from the public for over four decades, and a new study of historical documents finally revealed it.

For more information on this subject, check out the link below:

http://abcnews.go.com/Health/tobacco-companies-hid-evidence-radiation-cigarettes-decades/story?id=14635963

There is Ammonia in Coffee

A new invention relates to a process of treating coffee beans prior to domestic or institutional brewing of ground or roasted coffee. It forms a brew made from the coffee bean with lower acidity levels. This process gases the coffee bean with *ammonia gas* or *ammonium ions*. This lowers the level of acid in the coffee bean, making a better, less acidic brew of coffee.

There is ammonia in coffee—look at the link below:
http://www.sumobrain.com/patents/wipo/Process-preparation-deacidified-coffee/WO1996028038.html

What is Allergic Rhinitis?

"Allergic Rhinitis" a medical term for hay fever, (Rhinitis means "irritation of the nose" and is a derivative of rhino, meaning "nose"). Many substances cause the allergic symptoms that make up hay fever.

Symptoms include nasal congestion, a clear runny nose, sneezing, nose and eye itching, tearing eyes. Post-nasal dripping of clear mucus frequently causes a cough. Loss of smell is common and loss of taste occurs occasionally. Nose bleeding may occur if the condition is severe.

Ammonia is being overused and as a result, our mammals in the ocean are getting sick, this happens when ammonia gas fogs their minds and confuses the mammals and they beach themselves.

Ammonia poisoning is also linked with masses of bird dropping dead from the sky after air dropped ammonia chloride fertilizing was spread by a plane in farmer's fields.

To read more, check out the links below:

http://www.ehow.com/facts_6319581_ammoniaallergies.html#ixzz1o jbXD8v4

http://www.ehow.com/facts_6319581_ammonia-allergies.html#ixzz1ojbPdx45

http://symptoms.rightdiagnosis.com/cosymptoms/chronic-alzheimers-like-confusion-symptoms/elevated-blood-ammonia-level-all.htm

Chapter Six

What is Chloramine?

When ammonia and chlorine are combined together it makes a compound called "chloramine."

Chloramine is a hazardous chemical. Chloramine in our tap water can cause severe skin reactions like: rashes, dry skin, itching, welts, blisters, chapping, cracking, scarring, bleeding, flaking, and death.

It is lethal to fish, animals and humans. Six massive fish kills have been documented in the United States and Canada, killing everything in the reservoirs including the earthworms around the reservoirs.

They are using chloramine in reservoirs instead of chlorine in California and Connecticut and other states. Water companies across the United States are adding chlorine to their drinking water.

Chloramine can aggravate other skin conditions such as eczema and psoriasis. Chloramine can cause bleeding lips, dry mouth, and dry throat. Chloramine can cause burning, red, and dry eyes. Skin exposure to ammonia "breaks down cell structural proteins, extracts water from the cells, and initiates an inflammatory response, which further damages the surrounding tissues."

People in twenty states have reported respiratory problems, skin rashes, and digestive problems from drinking, cooking with, or bathing in chloraminated water.

The byproducts of chloramine are *100 TIMES MORE TOXIC* than those of chlorine. These byproducts are known to be damaging to DNA and to cells and can causing cancer.

Chloramine is *TWENTY THOUSAND TIMES LESS EFFECTIVE* in killing bacteria that cause water borne diseases.

Chloramine literally "eats rubber fittings in plumbing" and leaches lead into your children's water. Lead poisoning can cause developmental disabilities in children. The use of chloramine adds pollutants to the Chesapeake Bay and other watersheds and is destroying these bodies of water.

Digestive and Gastric Problems

Chloramine damages digestive mucosa. It can also aggravate digestive disorders. It is suggested that monochloramine is responsible for gastric cancer.

For an overview report on the development of gastric cancers in rats, click the link below for the PDF file report.

http://www.chloramine.org/articles_pdf/97_iishi_gastric_cancer_rats_r150.pdf

Kidney and Blood Problems

Persons with liver or kidney disease and those with hereditary urea cycle disorders are at increased risk for ammonia toxicity from the consumption of chloraminated water. Kidney dialysis patients cannot use chloraminated water in their dialysis machines because it will cause hemolytic anemia.

Chloramine must be completely removed from the water in dialysis treatment, using reverse osmosis filtering system and extensive carbon filtration to remove both chlorine and ammonia from the water. There are populations that are unusually susceptible to ammonia reactivity or toxicity due to factors such as genetic makeup, age, health status, etc.

Read more on this at:

http://www.chloramine.org/chloraminefacts.htm

http://www.thepetitionsite.com/2/stop-use-of-chloramine-in-drinking-water

Chapter Seven

How to Reduce Uric Acid in Your Body

In my research I found that natural, raw-unfiltered apple cider vinegar with mother (it will say "with mother" on the bottle label) does reduce uric acid in our bodies.

The mother of vinegar is actually a cellulose substance made up of various Acetobacter, a very acidic strain of bacteria. The Acetobacter combine with the oxygen in warm air to cause fermentation in apple cider, wine, or other alcoholic liquids to produce vinegar. It is the mother that gives the vinegar its characteristic sourness. There is also eleven percent potassium in apple cider vinegar with mother. This is normally strained out with the mother when clear apple cider vinegar is made.

Natural apple cider vinegar is made by crushing fresh, organically grown apples and allowing them to mature in wooden barrels. This boosts the natural fermentation qualities of the crushed apples, which differs from the refined and distilled vinegars found in supermarkets.

When the vinegar is mature, it contains dark, cloudy, web like bacterial foam called *mother*, which becomes visible when the rich brownish liquid is held to the light. The mother can be used to add to other vinegar to hasten maturity for making more apple cider vinegar.

Natural vinegars that contain the mother have enzymes, minerals, and natural yeast that other vinegars in grocery stores may not have due to over-processing, overheating, and filtration. For this reason, it is recommended that you purchase only *natural* apple cider vinegar, with an ideal acidity (pH) level of five to seven.

Apple cider vinegar that has been filtered and strained has no benefits, but it is good for salad dressing. You can get apple cider vinegar with the mother at your local health food store or sometimes your local grocery stores. I like the brand Bragg Organic Raw-Unfiltered Apple Cider Vinegar.

Check out their website at:

http://www.bragg.com/ It's full of information on apple cider vinegar.

To read more, check out the links below:

http://www.lacetoleather.com/wondrugpag3.html

http://www.homeremediesweb.com/apple_cider_vinegar_health_benefits.php

Chapter Eight

The History of Vinegar

Babylonians fermented date palm into vinegar as far back as 5,000 BC. Egyptian ruins dating back to 3,000 BC turn up vessels with vinegar remains in them. Early Greek and Roman artwork depict vinegar vessels in the scenery.

Hippocrates (fifth century BC) mentioned the health benefits of using vinegar to treat disease and infection, as well prescribing it as an overall elixir to balance the body's natural fluids (potassium also helps our cells maintain ideal fluid levels by acting as an electrolyte).

Claims

Over the years there have been many claims on the miracle of apple cider vinegar. One of the most popular is that drinking of apple cider vinegar each day will help you lose weight. However, it doesn't end there.

Many people also claim that it can kill head lice, reverse aging, wash the body of toxins, clear up hay fever, hiccups, menstrual problems, night sweats, hot flashes, helps with stomach digestion, gives you strong bones, clears up yeast infections, helps restore hair loss, insomnia, helps your nervousness and anxiety.

Many people also claim ACV clears up varicose veins, itchy scalp, headaches, dandruff, sunburn, acne, leg cramps, upset stomach, leg pain, asthma, cold, coughs, dizziness, fatigue, and migraines.

For a complete list, check out this website below for more:

http://www.naturalcurestome.com/apple-cider-vinegar.html

Throughout the millennia, in practically every global culture, vinegar has been used as an antiseptic, an energizing tonic, and a disease-prevention tonic as well as a condiment and flavoring.

Folks around the world as far back as Roman times have believed that raw vinegar can and does adjust your body's ph.

I found this out in my research: 100 mcg CHROMIUM is in apple cider vinegar with mother. The average American diet is deficient in chromium! Researchers estimate that two out of every three Americans are hypoglycemic or diabetic. The ability to maintain normal blood-sugar levels is jeopardized by the lack of chromium in our soil and water.

Chromium, an essential mineral, helps maintain stable blood-sugar levels. It is vital in the synthesis of fats, cholesterol, and proteins. It also vital in the metabolism of glucose, which is needed for energy, and it helps in the proper metabolism of amino acids. It promotes the loss of fat and an increase in lean muscle tissue.

To learn more click the link below:

http://www.webmd.com/diet/apple-cider-vinegar?page=2

They say apple cider vinegar can also be used topically to help reduce inflammation and pain. Around the world, people have consumed different varieties of raw vinegar for thousands of years, as not only a seasoning but also as a health tonic.

It is also being used as a topical soak for sunburns, itching, and yeast infections: Mix the vinegar and water in the form of one part vinegar to six parts cool or warm bathwater. Then soak the affected area for about thirty minutes and don't rinse off—just dry yourself off, then repeat as necessary.

Men for jock itch or foot fungus, Use both apple cider vinegar topical along with putting cornstarch on the infected areas after drying off. It clears up jock itch overnight—unless it's really bad; then it might take a little longer. Keep using cornstarch every day to stay clear from fungus, use cornstarch like powder between your legs.

Scientific Evidence

Very little research has been done on apple cider vinegar. This is pretty common for herbal remedies and supplements. After all, they don't need FDA approval in order to be sold, so many claims have not been researched as of yet.

ACV has long been promoted as a remedy for arthritis. The National Arthritis Foundation says apple cider vinegar has not been proven effective against arthritis but is harmless to try.

However, there have been a few studies done. Here is a list below:

1. **Diabetes:** Studies have shown that apple cider vinegar with mother reduces blood-sugar levels and reduces spikes in blood sugar.

2. **Weight loss:** Studies have shown that apple cider vinegar with mother and even white vinegar can aid in weight loss.

3. **Blood pressure and heart health:** Studies have also shown that apple cider vinegar with mother may reduce your blood pressure and help your heart health.

4. **High cholesterol:** Studies have shown that apple cider vinegar with mother reduces high cholesterol; however, these studies were done on mice and have never been done on people.

5. **Cancer:** Some research has been done on the use of apple cider vinegar with mother to treat cancer. However, these studies were also done on mice.

Chapter Nine

ACV Health Benefits

Apple cider vinegar (ACV) is one of the natural remedies I found to reduce uric acid in our bodies and keep our pH levels balanced. Some other natural remedies that also help to do this are herbs, fruits, and veggies.

ACV contains vitamins A, B1, B2, B6, C, and E, as well as beta-carotene and bioflavonoids. In addition to its excellent potassium supply, apple cider vinegar also contains trace minerals, including calcium, magnesium, phosphorus, boron, and sulfur—all important in the formation and maintenance of strong, dense bone structure.

Apple cider vinegar also contains tannins. Tannins are also found in tea, coffee, and red wine, as well as other fruits and vegetables, tannins are effective antioxidants. Raw apple cider vinegar is brimming with enzymes. Did you know that our bodies produce a number of enzymes naturally?

The rest of these powerful little digestive aids must be obtained from the foods we eat. Cooked foods have no enzyme activity at all. When food is heated, enzymes are lost. Raw foods contain some enzymes, but raw fermented foods like apple cider vinegar with mother are the most bountiful sources of enzymes.

Another nutritional reason why apple cider vinegar with mother is so good for us is that it is rich in potassium in an ideal dose for the human body. Potassium is an important mineral with many health benefits. Potassium acts like an electrolyte, which means that in the presence of sodium and chloride, it conducts electricity in the fluids of our bodies. Electrolytes are essential in allowing fluids into our cells and transporting waste products out.

Some enzymes require the presence of potassium in order to perform their functions. Potassium helps relieve muscle cramping, fatigue, and heart arrhythmia. It keeps our soft tissues (internal and external) soft and supple. This is important for *helping prevent hardening of the arteries.* Arteries are just one of the soft tissues in our bodies that benefit from apple cider vinegar with mother its potassium.

I also read people that have ECZEMA usually have a potassium deficiency. Apple cider vinegar has just the right dosage in it for our bodies. It's been reported that raw apple cider vinegar is good for helping reduce high blood pressure, most likely due to the potassium content.

Check out this web site:

http://www.organiccolorsystems.com/eczema-and-allergies/

Potassium also helps prevent tooth decay, splitting of fingernails, and hair loss, just to name a few more. Apple cider vinegar health benefits include its ability to return an overly acidic body to a more neutral pH level. Apple cider vinegar becomes naturally alkaline in your body, actually helping to counteract a hyper-acidity-body.

Pollution, environmental toxins, overconsumption of carbohydrates and refined sugars to name a few, all contribute to an overly acid body.

This doctor is tells us about the benefits of apple cider vinegar check out the link below:

http://www.healthdiaries.com/eatthis/10-health-benefits-of-apple-cider-vinegar.html

Apple Cider Vinegar with Mother

The Wonder "Drug"

Of

Yesterday,

Today

And

Tomorrow!

The Secret Fountain of Youth

Chapter Ten

What's in our Drinking Water?

It could be fluoride, chlorine and/or chloramine they are all acid based and used in our drinking water. Acid rots our teeth, and fluoride coats our teeth to keep them from rotting—or at least that's how it's supposed to work. But in large amounts, it's a poison to our bodies. The average consumer is not aware of the fluoride in their drinking water.

They are also not aware that sodium fluoride (**hydrofluosilicic** acid) is rated as more toxic than lead in chemistry indexes.

Read more on this at the link below:

http://www.justinandshannon.com/camp-keep-ocean/why-do-they-put-sodium-fluoride-in-our-water

Sodium Fluoride is a Poison

We don't know how much we are ingesting, so we don't know if we are being poisoned. No one knows the full extent or the long-term effects to fluoride buildup in our bones. Fluoride does cause pain, stiffness, and skeletal abnormalities in older people, that's because it is an accumulative poison. This pollutant has been collected in the phosphate fertilizer industry process.

Since sodium fluoride cannot be dump into our oceans, the government has allowed it to be dumped into our drinking water.

Sodium fluoride is a key component in anesthetic, hypnotic, and psychiatric drugs and sarin nerve gas.

Sodium fluoride is also one of the main ingredients in rat poison and it's in toothpaste and our drinking water.

Read more about this at:

http://search.yahoo.com/r/_ylt=A0oG7h6oBslP6FgAmmdXNyoA;_ylu=X3oDMTE1ODNoMWVzBHNlYwNzcgRwb3MDMwRjb2xvA2FjMgR2dGlkA01TWTAxM18xMjk/SIG=12ngiesvn/EXP=1338603304/**http%3a//home.vicnet.net.au/~fluoride/australian_fluoridation_faq.htm

Fluoride compounds where also added to the drinking water of prisoners in both Nazi prison camps during World War II and in the Soviet gulags in Siberia. They did it to keep the prisoners quiet and to control noncompliance with authority. Are they doing this to us also?

Must-read websites; please look at it you won't believe what you will read about ammonia and fluoride.

http://www.nrdc.org/water/pollution/cesspools/execsum.asp

http://fluoridedangers.blogspot.com/

Something else you need to know? I read that doctors tell us to drink at least eight glasses of water each day. Water is the most abundant chemical compound in living human cells, accounting for sixty five to ninety percent of each cell. That is why it is so important to drink water—it keeps flushing out that uric acid and other toxins that are in our bodies that are making us sick.

Read more on fluoride dangers:

http://www.purewatergazette.net/fluoride.htm

Don't drink tap water unless your home is equipped with a reverse-osmosis filtering system for its drinking water. Your city tap water has one or more of these chemicals lurking in it; fluoride, chlorine, and/or chloramine (ammonia & chlorine mixed together), and they are all acids and are *poison* to our bodies.

Our government has mandated putting fluoride in our drinking water why? Because the U.S. Public Health Service, (PHS) developed recommendations in the 1940s and 1950s regarding fluoride concentrations to be added in public water supplies to control cavities.

The Department of Health and Human Services has proposed a change to the recommended amount, of fluoride being put in out drinking water. Their proposal is to decrease the amount of fluoride from, 1.2 milligrams of fluoride per liter of water to 0.7 milligrams of fluoride per liter of water. This update will replace the recommendation provided in 1962 by the U.S. Public Health Service.

Check the labels on the bottled water you drink and make sure the water has gone through a reverse-osmosis filtering system; spring water is not filtered the same way as reverse-osmosis filtered water, and may still have dangers chemicals lurking in them. Also make sure there is no fluoride added. You may have to go to a health food store to buy water, but it's worth it.

You cannot eliminate all acids intake to your body that would be impossible to do because our bodies make a little bit of acid in our blood, and then converts it to uric acid. What I am trying to warn you from is all the man-made and unnecessary amounts of ammonia and other acids chemicals we put into our body each day.

One other thing you should think about doing as I mentioned above is to start drinking at least eight to ten glasses of water each day. That will keep flushing out that uric acid and also keep your body hydrated.

Many crops in this country are dusted with cryolite, a pesticide that contains energy-sapping fluoride. In January 2011, after being petitioned by health advocacy groups concerned about the harmful effects of too much fluoride, the Environmental Protection Agency announced plans to phase out cryolite. But the ban could take years to go into effect.

Until then, buying certain organic fruit and vegetables (especially tomatoes, strawberries, and potatoes, which have softer skins that can absorb more of the chemical) can help limit your exposure, says thyroid expert Richard Shames Md. In California many of the vineyards extensively use the pesticide on their grape crops, so when buying wine, consider sticking to varieties made in Europe, as cryolite is rarely used by winemakers there.

Read more at:

http://www.fluoridealert.org/

http://www.cdc.gov/fluoridation/fact_sheets/cwf_qa.htm

Fluoride is Lurking in Fresh Produce and Wine

Fluoride is found in toothpaste and in your water supply, every time you take a shower, brush your teeth, or drink from the tap, your body gets a little exposure to fluoride which leeches out good iodine from your body.

Read more here: http://search.yahoo.com/r/_ylt=A0oG7m25tNhPhQcAsgZXNyoA;_ylu=X3oDMTE1cGU4amhhBHNlYwNzcgRwb3MDMQRjb2xvA2FjMgR2d GlkA1ZJUDA5OV8xNTU-/SIG=12afvelb2/EXP=1339630905/**http%3a//www.naturalnews.com/031317_fluoride_iodine.html

Contrary to popular belief, fluoridated water is actually rather poor at preventing tooth decay.

Why is it in our water supply then? Poor science combined with corporate greed and political ignorance paved the way. Basically a toxic byproduct of aluminum production, fluoridation was sold as a way to prevent cavities.

This happened because some areas with natural fluoride in the water also had lower instances of tooth decay. Based upon that spurious observation, fluoridation began. (This comes from *WebMD*.)

According to the Centers for Disease Control and Prevention, only 2 mg of fluoride a day is needed to prevent tooth decay. Most of us get about three times that amount of fluoride, so cutting back won't hurt your teeth.

Check out this website to find out if your water has fluoride in it or if fluoride is added to it:

http://thyroid.org/patients/patient_brochures/iodine_deficiency.html

Iodine Deficiency

Iodine is a mineral, but one that is not abundant in the food we eat. Iodine deficiency affects about two billion people and is the leading

preventable cause of intellectual disabilities. While iodine is primarily found in very small quantities in seawater, soils are naturally deficient in it, especially the further away you get from the ocean. Iodine is also fairly easily displaced from your body by toxins called toxic halides—fluoride, bromine, and chloride.

Iodine deficiency is generally recognized as the most commonly preventable cause of mental retardation and the most common cause of end ocrinopathy (disorder in the function of an endocrine gland) (goiter and primary hypothyroidism).

Iodine deficiency becomes particularly critical in pregnancy, due to consequences for neurological damage during fetal development as well as the mother's milk during breast feeding period. Since iodine is an essential component of the thyroid hormone molecule, its deficiency during fetal development can cause hypothyroidism and irreversible mental retardation.

For more on this more on this check the link below:

http://thyroid.org/patients/brochures/IodineDeficiency_brochure.pdf

The Secret Fountain of Youth

Chapter Eleven

Other Things ACV is good for

It has also been suggested that apple cider vinegar reduces the craving for sweets and for foods containing salt and fat. *ACV acts as an appetite suppressant.* This is more than just a weight-loss theory—recent studies on raw vinegar as an appetite suppressant have been conducted by a team of Swedish scientists from Lund University. They have shown that raw vinegar taken in liquid form before a meal helps dieters eat less

According to Elin Ostman, "there is a direct relationship between increased acetic acid and hormone balance." For the studies, twelve healthy volunteers were given three amounts of vinegar (eighteen, twenty-three, and twenty-eight Mmol acetic acid—which is equal to about 1.5, 2, and 2.5 tablespoons of standard vinegar containing 5 percent acetic acid) diluted in water along with a portion of wheat bread containing fifty grams of available carbohydrate.

Satiety was measured with a subjective rating scale and was reported to be significantly increased at thirty, ninety, and a hundred twenty minutes after the meal. Apple cider vinegar was found to increases the body's metabolism thus burning more calories.

To read more on ACV as an appetite suppressant, from the European Journal of Clinical Nutrition, 2005, 59: 983-988. See the links below:

http://www.nature.com/ejcn/journal/v59/n9/abs/1602197a.html

http://www.apple-cider-vinegar-benefits.com/apple-cider-vinegar-history.html

The Secret Fountain of Youth

Chapter Twelve
The Secret Formula

I gave it a name:

Fountain Mist

Here is how you make Fountain Mist. Take one 16-ounce bottle of purified water; and drink about 2 ounces of the water to make room for the other ingredients. Add one tablespoon of apple cider vinegar with mother, add one package of bottle water flavoring, I like the punch flavor. (Its water bottle flavoring in a pouch,) I also like to add a pinch of baking soda to kill the acid, but you do not have to. Shake it up and sip or just drink it down—it's yummy!

I have one bottle of Fountain Mist in the morning, and one with my dinner. Check your pH often with alkaline test paper; use no more than six teaspoons of ACV a day, too much is not good either—find what works for your body, you might find just one bottle is fine for you. You can have up to two bottles of Fountain Mist a day.

Like many types of vinegar, apple cider vinegar with mother contains a substance called acetic acid. Apple cider vinegar with mother also contains some lactic, citric and malic acids. If you have any stomach pains check with your Doctor before drinking any more vinegar.

A famous Roman healer and philosopher Lucretius who understood the properties of vinegar and its health benefits more than two thousand years ago once said, "One man's food is another man's poison".

I did find some things about allergic reaction to ACV; it pertains to the acid if you take it straight out of the bottle without diluting it first in water, and do not take more then 2 tablespoons of ACV a day.

It's always a good practice to do an allergy test on anything new food going into your body. If you do get symptoms that make you uncomfortable and do not subside over time, try reducing the dose of ACV or discontinuing use it altogether, and talk to your Doctor about it.

Eat lots of alkaline foods and try to pick better food choices, when eat out at fast-food places. Eat very little food made with white flour; Nutritionist's telling us white flour is not good for us. They say eat food made with whole-wheat flour, and drink lots of water.

Here is some more good reading:

http://www.homeremediesweb.com/apple_cider_vinegar_health_benefits.php

http://www.apple-cider-vinegar-benefits.com/

Chapter Thirteen

Don't Panic

I started doing more researches to find out what could be causing so much sickness around me. I found out one of the things making us sick is, man-made ammonia—and it's everywhere and in almost everything we use. Some others dangerous chemicals are listed in this book also.

I wrote this book to help people understand what's happening to our planet and what could be making them sick. This is all connects to the global warming of the world. We all can do our part to correct this imbalance quicker, but we all have to do our part—not just pass the buck this time.

Ammonia gases are rising up into the sky causing global warming by deteriorating our ozone layer. Ammonia is also causing the oceans to have unusual growths like fungi and bryozoans. Scientist's claim it's not entirely clear why the fungi and bryozoans are appearing in such remarkable quantities.

Well it is now very clear: ammonia chloride is being poured into our oceans from our lakes, rivers, and sewer pipes. Ammonia and ammonium salts are also found in rainwater, whereas ammonium chloride (solution-ammoniac) and ammonium sulfate are found in volcanic districts.

Ammonium salts also are found distributed through all fertile soil and in seawater. And let's not forget the population of people around the world that's exploded, and the waste that comes from people that is also poured in to the oceans and in the ground.

I believe no one is keeping track of how much ammonia is really being used on our bodies, or in our bodies. I don't think anyone really knows how much is too much for our bodies to handle before we get sick. I cannot find on the Web, any studies that have been done on people or animals with ammonia. Not even tests showing ammonia is safe for human consumption or safe levels for human consumption. I can only find how bad ammonia can be to us if we get over exposure to ammonia and how much was being produced around the world.

Because of its many uses, ammonia is one of the most highly produced organic chemicals in the world. This is just something that happened as our population grew and food demands changed. New, wonderful products were developed like the refrigerators and freezers, which use ammonia to keep them cold.

We all welcomed A/C in our cars and in our homes. Everyone likes using these things, but they use Freon gas, which Is ammonia. There has been a change in using ammonia as a refrigerant for residential and auto use, but it's still being use commercially. As our ammonia demands grew, new businesses spring up and started using ammonia. Supply and demand for ammonia are being met but at what cost.

As the world population grows our landfills are get bigger, and we dump more grass clippings, septic tank waste, food scraps, wood, silicone, paint, metal, plastic and all kinds of acids in the landfills year after year, and it's fermenting and making methane gas. Ammonia is now building up in the form of methane gas (ammonia gas) and going up to the ozone layer and helping to deplete it.

Dozens of chemical plants worldwide produce ammonia. The worldwide man-made ammonia production in 2004 was 109 million metric tons. China produced 28.4 percent of that worldwide production from coal as part of urea synthesis), followed by India with 8.6 percent, Russia with 8.4 percent, and the United States with 8.2 percent.

About 80 percent or more of the ammonia produced is used for fertilizing agricultural crops. In 2006, worldwide production was estimated at 146.5 million tons. In 20there was a numerous of large-scale ammonia production plants worldwide, producing a total of 131,000,000 metric tons of ammonia.

We will always need honest doctors, because not all sickness comes from chemical poisoning and there will always be those that won't listen and will refuse to take apple cider vinegar with mother for one reason or another.

Because most people won't do anything after reading this book except continue to do what they have already done. So even though I have uncovered some chemicals that are making us sick, and killing us slowly, the doctors, the FDA, and the pharmaceutical industry will never go out of business; they are much needed and so are the good drugs they make.

http://www.ccohs.ca/oshanswers/chemicals/chem_profiles/ammonia/health_ammonia.html

http://www.buzzle.com/articles/anhydrous-ammonia-fertilizers.html

Chapter Fourteen

In Closing

Keep your pH levels between 7.0 and 7.2 this is perfect pH for your body. Below 6.9 is too acidic and above 7.5 is too alkaline for your body.

I have a question for you: after reading this book, did you come up with the same conclusion I did?

If you start using *Fountain Mist*, I would like to know how you are feeling after your first week, first month, first three months, first six months, and first year. Tell me what pains are gone from your body, and if your movement is better. I really want to know. Also let me know, are you getting sick less often, and is your mind clearer and you're overall health?

I may writing a follow-up book and I may use some of the feedback you e-mail me, without using your name. My e-mail address is calljons@gmail.com.

THANK YOU FOR READING MY BOOK

~JON MICHAEL CARAVELLA~

DISCLAIMER: DUE TO THE LACK OF SUPPORTING RESEARCH BY OUR GOVERNMENT, THE FOOD AND DRUG ADMINISTRATION, AND THE AMERICAN MEDICAL SOCIETY FOR SPORTS MEDICINE, APPLE CIDER VINEGAR CANNOT BE RECOMMENDED FOR TREATMENT OR PREVENTION OF ANY HEALTH PROBLEMS. ALSO, PLEASE CONSULT WITH YOUR PHYSICIAN, PHARMACIST, OR HEALTH-CARE PROVIDER BEFORE TAKING ANY HOME REMEDIES OR SUPPLEMENTS. I'M JUST SHARING MY EXPERIENCE AND WHAT WORKS FOR ME AND FOR THOUSANDS OF OTHERS I HAVE READ ABOUT.

To keep the record straight with the FDA and our Government, I must say this. I am not a doctor but I am a researcher and a writer. Everything in this book I found on the World Wide Web. I have made up nothing except the name *Fountain Mist for my drink*.